REFLEXOLOGY TODAY

A guide to the theory and practice of reflexology — the art of restoring the body to health through special massage techniques applied to the feet.

D0210325

REFLEXOLOGY TODAY

The Stimulation of the Body's Healing Forces Through Foot Massage

by

Doreen E. Bayly

THORSONS PUBLISHERS LIMITED
Wellingborough, Northamptonshire

First edition published in 1978 by Doreen E. Bayly
This revised edition published 1982
Fifth Impression 1985

British Library Cataloguing in Publication Data

Bayly, Doreen E.
    Reflexology today.—2nd ed.
    1. Reflexotherapy 2. Massage 3. Foot
    I. Title
    615.8'22   RM723.R43

    ISBN 0-7225-0705-4

Printed and bound in Great Britain

Contents

ACKNOWLEDGEMENTS

I wish to express my grateful thanks to all those who have so patiently helped me to prepare this book for publication.

Also my thanks to Alan Raddon for his help in designing the line drawings and assembling the illustrations; to M.J. Vukovic and Ian Dawson for the photographs.

DEDICATED TO
the memory of Rowena Mummery for
her help and inspiration.

Preface to First Edition

In response to many urgent requests for a book on the therapy of reflexology, I am publishing my experiences in pioneering the work in Great Britain since training under Miss Eunice D. Ingham in America. During this time, careful study and observation has been made of cases and the results obtained by the skilful application of the therapy on a great many patients. A large reserve of knowledge was thus accumulated before I took the franchise licence to teach.

My experience when I returned to England in 1966 was to find that people regarded the subject with complete indifference. This was something of a shock after the eagerness shown for the treatment by the people in America. Some months passed by before even one pair of feet was entrusted to my hands.

When some new treatment is introduced and the word spread by recommendation the progress is often slow, since the results have to justify the claims made for it. But success comes to all good things in time, and today it is gratifying to know that my students are practising in large numbers in Great Britain and on the Continent. In fact, they have spread world-wide.

All information given in this book on the theory and practice of reflexology, and the resulting health benefits is based on my own experiences and is offered to all serious students who wish to practise correctly, so that they can give the greatest help to others and to themselves.

I hope that the large numbers of people who have appealed to me to write this book will find all that they wish to know concerning the technique of reflexology, and that it will be a book of reference to which they can always turn when in doubt about how to treat a certain condition. With this in mind, there is a section given over to case histories of people who have been treated by me, and although these are brief, I hope that the information given will help students decide how best to treat any similar case.

Any reference to another authority is always acknowledged by name and source.

Doreen E. Bayly
London, February 1978

Introduction

Now that public interest has been aroused in the subject of treating disorders of the body through the reflexes, books on the subject are coming onto the market all the time. Some information is far from accurate, verging on the realm of chimera. I believe that it is necessary for a book to be written giving a clear and commonsense description of how reflexology works, and the range of disorders that can be treated by its use. My writing is based on years of experience and is not a rehash of the writings of others. The high rate of success is empirical and not based on vague and untested theories.

The aim of this book is to give the student and public alike a clear understanding of reflexology, how it works, and why it differs from other therapies. The scope of the work and its all-embracing range of benefits is remarkable. By massage given on the reflexes of the feet an increase in the blood circulation takes place. Tension is also relaxed throughout the nervous system. This releases the strain under which the body is suffering, which restores the normal energy flow. Thus the body is gradually brought back to the normal balance that is necessary for perfect health.

Reflexology is not a 'cure-all' but a means of helping the body attain perfect balance in all its functions in every system. It is all-embracing fundamentally because it influences the whole area where weakened circulation has allowed waste matter to interfere with the free flow of vital forces necessary to life. The whole body is encouraged to renew itself so that all its processes are working in harmony. Massage of the reflexes of the feet will bring about a stimulation of the healing forces that are latent in the body, and by working upon the various systems – circulatory, glandular, and nervous – much can be done to normalize the functions operating throughout the whole organism.

Reflexology is also of the greatest use as a means of diagnosis. It is fantastic for this purpose: it is quickly applied and is accurate. By testing the various reflexes in the feet, the degree of tenderness will give an accurate reading of any organ or area that is in a state of disorder.

The study of reflexology is based on a knowledge of anatomy and physiology. For those who have little or no knowledge of the functions of the body, further study is essential in order to use the reflex method to its full capacity. It is advisable to start on some basic text books and then move on to more advanced works later. So much knowledge has been accumulated about the human body in all aspects of health and disease, and so vast are the number of volumes written about it that it is difficult for the student to decide which medical books to study. The study of reflexology can begin from the time when the student reads this book and starts to practise on a pair of feet. As the student acquires greater knowledge of the human body, his work will become more competent.

Working as a reflexologist is a fascinating experience; so quickly do the results show, often whilst the treatment is being given. A person may come for treatment looking depressed and tired, but as the massage is given upon the feet and the circulation improves, together with the relaxing of tension, the whole attitude of the person changes. The face will show a glow of returning vitality and by this change it can be seen that the work has started to restore the depleted energies, even though it may be necessary to give several more treatments to complete the relief of the condition.

No limit can be laid down as to the number of treatments needed; this will vary according to the type of disorder and the length of time it has been suffered. Usually the trouble yields more quickly when it is of recent origin. It has to be remembered that damaged or weak tissue has to be replaced as the body is stimulated by the therapy, and where much repair is needed, the time of recovery will be longer.

If we look briefly at the basic processes by which the life force of a living organism operates, we see that the billions of cells of which it is composed are in a constant state of growth and decay. In the growing organism the formation of cells must be greater than the destruction of cells. For health, the growth of cells must equal the death of cells. In maturity the balance between the two must be maintained. When the body loses the ability to maintain this balance, the entire structure ages. The work of reflexology can do much to arrest the ageing process, by stimulating the nerve and vascular systems, and so ensuring a better blood supply.

Large versions of the charts illustrated at the back of this book can be obtained from:

Crusade Against All Cruelty to Animals Limited,
Humane Education Centre, Avenue Lodge,
Bounds Green Road, London N22 4EU
Tel: 01-889 1595

Please send s.a.e. for price list.

1. What is Reflexology?

The questions 'What is reflexology?' and 'What are the processes that take place in the body?' are queries for which various explanations have been put forward in answer. Quite probably two or three processes are brought into operation by the use of compression massage which contribute to the remarkable results obtained. Undoubtedly there is still much to learn about the restoration of health through the stimulation of certain areas of the feet when deep massage is applied.

The breaking up and dispersing of crystals which are deposited in the reflexes, interfering with blood circulation and causing congestion, is the usual theory put forward about what actually happens. There is also, I believe, an electrical impulse triggered off by pressure massage on a tender reflex and there is the subtle energy flow which brings that remarkable return of vitality to the patient even while receiving treatment. This varies with the sensitivity of the individual.

I believe the electrical impulse acts on the body in the same way that the stimulus of light acts on the retina of the eye. Dr John N. Ott of the Roswell Park Memorial Institute, Center for Light Research in Buffalo, New York, together with other scientists, has done much research on the effect of light upon the body. It has been proved that the action of the full spectrum of light on the retina of the eye, in which are embedded the endings of the optic nerve, produces an electrical impulse which is carried to the hypothalamus, from whence it is passed down to the pituitary gland, which passes down to the lesser glands, thereby activating all the functions of the body. It is my belief that the work upon the reflexes produces similar results.

I have the permission of Dr John Ott to quote from his findings on the effect of light on laboratory mice with cancer tumours. It was found that mice kept under artificial light developed tumours two to three months earlier than mice kept under natural daylight. One can assume that the strong impulse registered on the eyes definitely assisted in retarding the cancer development. With regard to the subtle vitality flow, this links with the etheric part of man bringing about a harmony between the etheric and the physical bodies. I talked, not long ago, with a well-known biologist who is one of the foremost authorities on the lymphatic system. He holds the theory that the spiritual energy travels through the interstitial fluid of the lymphatic system to flood the whole organism.

There is still much to discover, but we know that we have in our hands a wonderful therapy, one which will be developed as one of the most important methods of natural healing of the future.

2. The Structure of the Feet

The foot is a wonder of engineering. The bones are so formed that they combine great strength with a fine degree of flexibility. I beg all of you who are working on the feet to give time to the study of their anatomy.

The tarsus is formed of seven bones, one of which, the talus, takes the thrust of the body's weight from the tibia and fibula in the leg and distributes it between the heel and the tarsal bones, which then shift the weight on to the metatarsals and phalanges. Because of the number of these bones (there are nineteen of them) they give great pliability and strength.

The sole is composed of layers of tough fibrous muscles and ligaments, the chief being the long plantar. Bands of muscle traverse and bind together these layers in a wonderful way. The plantar artery rises in the top of the foot to become the plantar arch and from it branch smaller arteries to carry the blood supply to each toe. The foot is also well supplied with nerves and lymphatic glands.

When treating the feet it is necessary to give sufficient pressure to bring about results, but rough heavy probing given ruthlessly over a period of time negates the principle of the work. Miss Eunice Ingham once said to me, 'If you work on the reflex too long, you are undoing the good you have done.' It used to be said that a weary horse if beaten continually would in the end be too exhausted to respond to the punishment. We can here draw a parallel with the danger of overdoing the work. One of my students told of a case, which is mentioned elsewhere in this book, of a woman who developed an abscess in the breast through a severe injury to the breast reflex on the foot. Therefore rough treatment of a reflex must be liable to cause distress to the organ being treated.

I advise the treatment be given for about half an hour. Sore reflexes should get extra attention, but if the tenderness does not yield after some minutes of massage, it is best to discontinue and give the sore reflexes extra treatment on the next visit.

Another thing to be remembered is that feet do vary in texture and sensitivity. A highly strung person will often have a rather thin type of foot and will respond much more quickly to reflex pressure than someone more phlegmatic with a plump foot and deeper reflexes. We must always be ready to think and decide what is best for each individual. We need to be alert and responsive to the clues given by the reaction to pressure on the reflexes of the feet.

The Zones and Cross Reflexes

First the zones must be studied and memorized (see chart at back of book). Within their framework we locate the areas to be worked upon. The zones are lines running the entire length of the body. There are five on each side of the medial line. On either side of the middle or medial line is zone one, then passing over to the side of the body are zones two, three, four and five. Again, on the arms and legs the zones are repeated. Number one running down to the thumb, out to five on the little finger. In the legs and feet the zoning is the same. It is within these zones that the energy flow links the organs in that zone. If one area is out of order the whole of the zone may be affected. Sometimes the pain will manifest at a distance from its origin, having been referred to another part of the zone.

The hands have the same reflexes as the feet, but they are not quite so clearly defined because the hands are so much more mobile than the feet which are confined in shoes. However, the ability to work on the hands must always be remembered, and is most important when for some reason the feet cannot be treated. In cases of injury or amputation of a foot, great relief can still be given through the hands. Also in cases where elderly people cannot reach their feet, it is possible for them to help relieve various pains by using the knowledge of the hand reflexes. I have known many such cases.

There is another set of cross reflexes which are most important. These are between the shoulder and the hip, and the elbow and the knee. These cross reflexes should always be remembered and used when necessary. The results will be quite remarkable. In the course of my work I have seen cases where, owing to a painful injury on the foot, the hand and arm on the same side have become extremely painful owing to the sympathetic connection between the hand and the foot. By using the cross method of massage, rapid relief can be given.

One of the many cases which responded to the method was that of a lady who had fallen and sustained a Colles' fracture of the wrist. She had been to hospital and the fracture had been set and put into plaster. When she returned home she was in extreme pain and she sent for me. I arrived and immediately looked at the ankle on the same side of the body as the fractured wrist. I found, as I expected, that the ankle was swollen and very tender. This was due to the sympathetic reaction between the ankle and the wrist. Reflex massage was given to the foot with thorough massage to the ankle area. Results were good. The pain was relieved in the hand and wrist, and the tenderness also disappeared from the ankle.

Always remember that so often a condition can be relieved by using the knowledge of the cross reflexes to speed recovery. When studying reflexology always get thoroughly acquainted with the framework of the zones and cross reflexes. They give the background for your success (see chart).

3. How to Give a Treatment

The comfort of the patient is all important. A reclining chair offers the ideal position for a person receiving treatment. Should a treatment couch have to be used, a pillow must be placed under the head and another under the knees. The room must be warm. In the case of a woman wearing a skirt, a towel should be used to cover the legs because loss of heat causes the body to become more tense and relaxation is essential.

If visiting people in their own homes, you may have to improvise. An armchair will be quite adequate, with a stool or another chair for the legs. You should sit on a low chair or stool, if possible, to work on the feet.

You will learn from experience that it is important to gain a person's confidence. Ask if discomfort is felt when certain areas are pressed upon, also how long the disorder has been giving distress. Explain that the answers to such questions can help you diagnose which organs are in trouble, and that the health may soon improve with a course of treatment.

Take the right foot in your hands and start to massage the big toe. You will have studied the charts and know that the toes contain the reflexes to the head. Try to visualize that the two feet placed together represent the human body, even though of a different shape. With a corner of your thumb press into the tissues to find the tender reflex which is only a small area. Your movement combines both pressure and massage.

Both the thumb and the fingers can be used (thumb- and finger-nails should be short) for compression massage, but it is best to use the thumb whenever possible. As you work over the soles of the feet and locate the reflexes, the degree of discomfort must be noted. Also be attentive to the amount of pressure needed to get a response on the reflex.

The movement is not easily acquired. To reach a stage of full proficiency, training at a reflexology seminar under a qualified practitioner is necessary. Feet differ in texture to a great extent, and varying pressures are needed. Training and careful observation give the experience and sensitivity needed for obtaining the best results.

The timing of a treatment is important, because enough massage must be given but not too much. At the first treatment the time should be about twenty minutes. The reaction felt by the patient should be noted, if any. Usually tiredness is felt the next day because the body has been stimulated to throw off waste matter into the blood stream. Upon the next treatment the time can be lengthened to thirty minutes — that is fifteen minutes to each foot. Each reflex should be checked over and those that are very tender must receive a few minutes extra massage. Gradually the soreness will become less and the practitioner may then move on to another area. Always, if possible, give the relaxing exercise at the end. This consists of pressing upon the solar plexus reflex and moving the feet in unison with the patient's slow breathing. This exercise is taught at every seminar.

When Not to Give Treatment

Reflexology is a remarkably safe therapy, but there are times when it is advisable to be careful in its application.

It is important to remember when treating children that a very different pressure should be used, much lighter than the pressure given to adults. For a very young baby of a few weeks old it is enough to use one finger and gently stroke the feet. As children grow older greater pressure may be used and the practitioner must use his own judgment. For a girl approaching puberty, again care must be taken. At this time the glandular system is in a state of heightened activity, and over-excitement is not wise.

I had a student who went home after the first day of class that she was attending and treated her little girl, who was about ten years old, I believe. She found the child's reflexes very tender, especially those of the kidney, ureter tube, and bladder. Being under the impression that all sore areas must be worked upon until the tenderness disappeared, she worked much too long upon them. She should have realized that the condition was due to the child's age. As it was, she sent her to bed and she became incontinent during the night, due, of course, to the over-stimulation she had received. I also know of one case where harshly applied reflex treatment at the commencement of menstruation resulted in the period becoming almost continuous throughout the four week cycle.

Remember that all children's feet are far more responsive to our work than adults', so treat accordingly.

Remember that cases of chronic heart trouble should be treated with care upon the heart reflex until the condition of the whole body has responded to the work and the muscle tone has been helped by continued treatment upon the adrenals and all other endocrine glands.

Remember that if asked to treat a case of thrombosis the consent of the doctor in charge of the case should be obtained. The doctor may not wish any form of stimulation to be given.

4. The Glands

A student put the question to me not long ago: 'Why do you talk so much about the glands and soft organs of the body instead of the skeletal system?' My answer was that the whole body depends upon the blood to live. No part of the body can survive as a living part without the blood being carried into the bone through the nutrient foramen to feed the cancellous tissue. The glands depend upon the blood supply, and the blood depends upon the correct functioning of the glands in return: so intricate are the processes going on within the organism. The glandular system is all important. The secretions produced by the glands are many and varied and vital to life. Some are little known even now.

The Pituitary Gland
The pituitary stands first and foremost amongst the glands and controls the whole glandular system. It is the first cell to

be formed at conception. For this reason it is called the Master Gland. It is situated in the centre of the head and at the base of the brain in a depression known as the sella turcica of the sphenoid bone. The size of the gland is only that of a pea, yet it is divided into two lobes, each of which secretes hormones with different functions. It is overshadowed by the hypothalamus through which the secretions of the pituitary are controlled.

The Thyroid Gland
The thyroid gland is under the control of the pituitary. The thyroid in turn controls the lesser glands, and is responsible for growth, energy and clear thinking. The thyroid also has a close link with the reproductive organs.

The Parathyroid Glands
These are small endocrine glands which control the calcium distribution in the body. There are four of these, situated upon the posterior aspect of the thyroid. PTH, the hormone produced by the parathyroid glands regulates the calcium content of the body and its distribution to various organs. Should the glands become diseased and unable to function, the bones may become softened and collapse. If the parathyroid glands should be removed during thyroid surgery, tetany spasm will occur, and this can be dangerous if immediate treatment is not given. The parathyroids, if out of balance, are responsible for the incidence of arthritis, to a large extent.

The Pancreas
The gland lies across the midline of the body and secretes enzymes for the digestion of the contents of the small intestine. It also produces the hormone insulin in the Langerhans' islets. Should the hormone not be produced, then diabetes mellitus which is often called sugar diabetes will develop.

The Adrenals (Suprarenal Glands)
The glands are situated on the top of the kidneys secreting adrenalin from the suprarenal medulla. Cortisone is produced by the adrenal cortex. The glandular secretions are responsible for muscle tone, energy, and growth.

The Gonads
The male testicles produce semen and secrete hormones which promote growth and secondary sexual development.

The female ovaries produce ova and hormones which control sexual development and oestrogen to regulate the menstrual cycle.

5. Disorders to be Treated Through the Big Toe

Migraine
This condition may have several causes:

Occupational. When working under stress, or doing work involving eye strain or tension in the occipital and cervical areas of the head and neck, migraine may become an occupational hazard.

Liver condition causing a poor elimination of bile. Diet

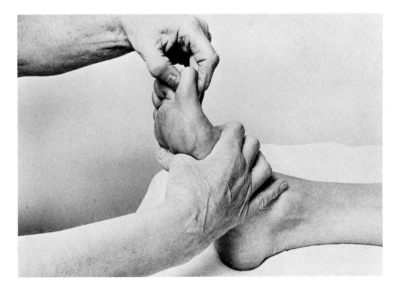

The pituitary reflex

often plays a big part in this condition. Too large an intake of fats may aggravate it. Food allergies may also trigger off an attack.

Tension caused by a highly nervous temperament. Menstrual difficulties may bring on an attack for some women.

Treatment
Reflex massage on the big toe, working on the inside and also on the outside, especially the area on the outside and the neck area of the toes to relieve the tension on the cervical reflex. Attention should be given to the liver reflex and the colon reflex. It is very important to treat the solar plexus to relax the patient. A general treatment should also be given to balance the body and to tone it.

Polio
It is believed that the paralysis which follows an attack of poliomyelitis is caused by the damage done to the pituitary gland during the attack. The severe imbalance of the gland upsets the lesser glands under its control. Miss Eunice Ingham claimed that when treating such cases she found

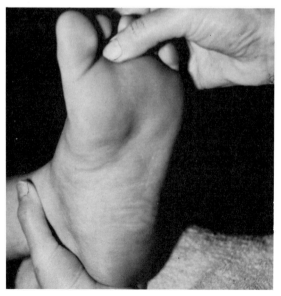

The eye reflex

the greatest degree of tenderness to be always in the reflex to the pituitary. She helped many young people back on to their feet again with her work. I have recently seen improvement in cases where the polio attacked over twenty years before.

Treatment
Give a general treatment to help the body regain its normal balance and full blood supply to all parts, but always work on and give all the massage possible to the pituitary reflex. Also pay great attention to the whole length of the spinal reflex, and always treat the colon reflex to ensure healthy elimination.

Eyes
Treatment for eye disorders is given at the base of the toes: zones two and three. Massage should be given below the toes. Tenderness should be noted, and if the painful area is close to the big toe, it may indicate inflammation in the tearduct.

Glaucoma is a disorder that will usually respond to treatment. In some cases the pressure in the eyeball will drop to normal after a course of treatment. Of course it depends on how long the person has suffered with the trouble, and should an operation have been performed the condition will be slow to yield. Always work on the kidney reflexes which are in the same zone as the eyes. The trouble may be aggravated by the faulty functioning of the kidneys, causing excessive acid in the body.

The Optic Nerve. The optic nerve has its origin in the hypothalamus and extends to the back of the eye. The nerve ends are embedded in the retina. Various conditions may affect the full functioning of the nerve, such as a heavy blow on the head or a fall causing severe jarring to the head and neck. Kidney disorders, and even the pressure from ingrowing toenails may seriously interfere with the optic nerve reflex. Massage should be given to the eye reflex, also to the head and cervical reflexes. There have been many remarkable recoveries recorded. I have myself treated such cases with great success.

Cataract. In many cases cataract can be helped by reflexology massage given over a period of time, with special attention to the reflexes of the kidneys and colon. I believe the condition to be aggravated by food deficiencies, so it is well to advise old people to take vitamin supplements for additional nourishment as they are particularly prone to this disorder.

One of my cases was a woman over ninety years old. She responded with a degree of improvement in her vision which continued until, through extreme age, the sight failed with her general health at the end of her life.

Reflexology can be used to improve a person's general health so that after undergoing an operation they are so fit that they quickly recover. One such case was a lady suffering from cataract that was due for surgery who had wisely decided upon a course of reflex therapy. Although she was over eighty years of age, she came through the experience with flying colours. Afterwards she expressed surprise at feeling so well, saying that she was feeling better than she had done for years.

Treatment
Massage the eye reflex once or twice a week and always follow with a general treatment over the whole of both feet. Any tenderness in the area of the small intestines and the colon should be carefully worked upon. The kidneys also must never be forgotten, because the general health of the whole body is all important.

Ears
Deafness will yield to treatment in some cases but not in others. If there is a large amount of scar tissue, due possibly to surgery, or an accident, the condition will only improve to a certain extent. If the deafness is due to a nerve condition, then help can be given by improving the general health through a course of treatment to the whole of the feet. Special attention to the cervical area of the spinal reflex will relieve tension at the back of the neck. Worry, with the resulting tension, and also excessive tiredness, will increase this type of deafness.

Another disorder which contributes to deafness is a catarrhal infection of the Eustachian tube. The reflex is between the reflexes of the eye and the ear. It will be found to be extremely tender if an infection is present.

Injuries to the Head

Cases of severe pain resulting from concussion, skull fracture, or severe laceration which has caused much scar tissue to form can be given tremendous relief by a course of treatment. If the case is one where the injury occurred several years before, the treatment will have to be given for some time to relax the scar tissue. I had a case of a woman who had received a severe concussion when in her teens which had resulted in continual pain (see patient's own story in Appendix). The headache reached unbearable intensity at times. She was in middle age when she came for help. Treatment was given over a period of time. At first there were only short periods of ease from the pain, but as the massage continued with weekly treatments, the pain became gradually less, and the pain-free periods grew longer until she eventually recovered.

A point to remember when treating cases of head injury: always check for ingrown toenails. This lady was advised to ask her chiropodist to correct the nails and remove any pressure. The improvement was immediate. Constant pressure from the nail interferes with the pituitary reflex. There are many cases of such conditions on record where great relief has been given through the application of careful chiropody.

Cerebral Haemorrhage

This is a condition where a blood vessel in the brain has ruptured. The cause is usually high blood pressure with hardening of the arteries. Sometimes low blood pressure can be to blame. Severe tension in the solar plexus brought on by worry and mental tension also contributes. Sometimes imbalance of the body induced by an unhealthy colon or poorly functioning kidneys may cause calcium deposits to form.

Treatment by working on the reflexes of the feet should be given as quickly as possible. I have had remarkable results, and there are many cases on record of treatment given by other practitioners with great success. By giving compression massage on both big toes as well as other important areas, help is given to keep the blood circulating, and so carry oxygen to the brain cells which so quickly die without oxygen. If help is given without delay, the patient will not only show signs of recovery, but paralysis will be prevented.

Treatment

Work on both toes on the brain area and the pituitary reflex. The area for the cervicals must be massaged to prevent tension building up at the back of the neck. The heart reflex needs massage to help the heart overcome the strain imposed on it. The solar plexus reflex should receive special attention to relax tension and quieten the patient. I have seen a patient recover the power of speech and able to focus the eyes in twenty minutes when reflex massage was used on the feet. The patient had just gone down with a stroke. Do always remember that everything possible should be done, talking reassuringly to the patient, who may be aware of his condition but unable to speak. Also **do not** discuss the patient's condition with another person within earshot of the patient: hearing is often the last sense to be affected.

In cases where the stroke has occurred some time before, the same type of treatment should be given, with massage over the whole foot and extra massage to the adrenal reflexes, to help the muscle tone and aid the body to restore the wasted tissues. The patient must be encouraged to strive to make all possible movement. Sometimes recovery is a slow affair.

(For further details of the foregoing cases, please refer to the case histories at the end of this book.)

6. The Spinal Reflex

A very important part of the foot treatment is the spinal reflex. The spine can be looked upon as an extension of the brain. The nerves carry impulses from all parts of the body through the spine to the brain. The spine conveys impulses from the brain which direct and control all functions, throughout the body.

After working on the big toes it is a good idea to treat the length of the spinal reflex and note any tender areas.

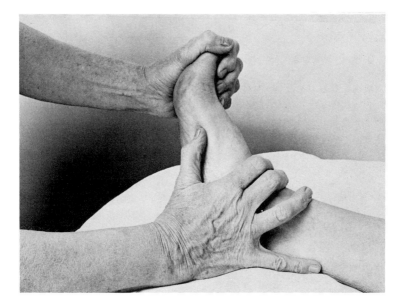

Position for massaging the spinal reflex

These may be of great use when making an assessment of the patient's condition. Old injuries, possibly of many years' standing, will show up and link with the disorder being treated. Remember that there is a peculiar link between the head and the coccyx. Sometimes a headache will be relieved by working on the reflex area of the coccyx, which may have been injured long before. When traversing the spinal reflex with the thumb, check for variations of the line of the reflex, because in some people it will be on the side of the foot and in others it will be almost underneath – on the sole.

The majority of patients come with spinal trouble and they respond to treatment in a remarkable way. In some cases of longstanding pain due to wounds, or other injury, I have been able to bring about a complete recovery from pain and stiffness, even after many years. Often after a car accident the spine has 'buckled', causing a lateral curvature. In these cases a great degree of relief can be given to the tension present and even an amount of straightening as the tension is released.

7. The Importance of the Thyroid and Parathyroid

The thyroid gland is a two-lobed organ which lies in front of the trachea and flanks it on either side. Its functions are of the greatest importance. Any state of imbalance in the thyroid brings distress. Its secretion is thyroxin, which controls metabolism, growth, and sexual development.

Hypersecretion creates hyperthyroidism
    (1) elevated heart action
    (2) elevated exophthalmic condition

Hyposecretion creates:
    (1) goitre – enlarged gland
    (2) hypothyroidism (cretinism) myxoedema
    (3) (a) low heart rate and blood pressure
          (b) low body temperature.
Reflexology treatment, because it works to relieve the

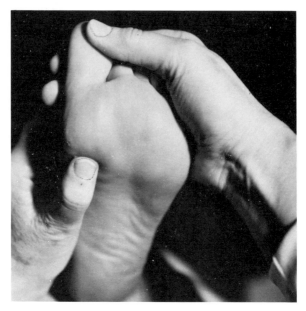

Massage on the thyroid reflex

fundamental cause of the disorder, can help the body to regain the correct balance. So whether the function of the thyroid be over- or under-active, the treatment will be of great value in restoring a normal condition. Always massage deeply into the prominence below the big toe when treating for thyroid disturbance, noting the parts that are the most tender. The full functioning of the thyroid is dependent upon the full intake of oxygen by the lungs for a maximum performance. Thus once again it is brought to our notice how interdependent one organ is upon another if all is to work in harmony.

Do not forget the close link between the reproductive organs and the thyroid. Always work on the reflexes to the ovary or testicle reflex, then follow up with treatment on the thyroid reflex. The cells forming the structure of both the reproductive organs and the thyroid are said to be of similar type and there is a very intimate link between them at all times. The thyroid is also of the same type of tissue as that of the pituitary gland.

One case of mine was a woman of about fifty years who came to me because of long-standing thyroid trouble. At the age of eighteen she had been operated on because of over-activity in the gland. Evidently too much of the gland was removed and the whole of her metabolism was affected. She became slow and depressed, developing a malignancy of the uterus in middle life. Surgery for this was successful, and there was no return of the disease. Her appearance was one of great weakness. Her skin colour was poor, she was over-weight, and she moved slowly. She complained of constant pressure on the top of her head as though she carried a weight there. As she had a very responsible job she was unable to undergo prolonged reflexology treatment, but she booked for eight visits in advance. From the first treatment her condition improved. She said the pressure on her head was relieved at once. She became brighter, more active and the depression left her. At the end of eight treatments she said that she was feeling fine. From time to time in the ensuing two years contact was made and she always replied: 'I am fine and so grateful for the help given.'

Parathyroids

Always remember what an important role the parathyroids

play in the body metabolism. Calcium, phosphate, magnesium and citrate ions (molecules carrying an electrical charge) keep body processes in balance, and each has a vital function to perform. They are carried in the extra-cellular fluid (plasma, interstitial fluid). These substances are essential to bone, muscle formation and energy production. The regulation of the cellular and fluid level of calcium in the body is under the primary control of the parathyroid glands.

Never forget to massage the parathyroid reflexes when giving treatment in cases of arthritis.

8. The Head

The study of the body in relation to applying the reflex therapy must start with the head. It is all important: holding the brain which controls the whole of the body and is the seat of consciousness. It will therefore be understood that

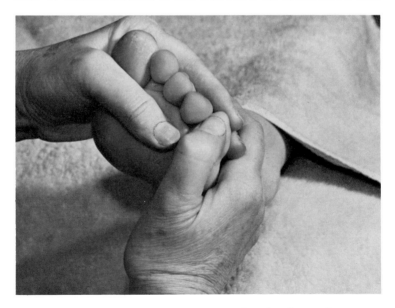

How to hold the foot when massaging the sinus reflex

when a treatment by compression massage is given, because the toes contain the reflexes to the head, they are the first parts to be treated. The big toes represent the brain area. The small toes relate to the sinuses of the frontal and nasal cavities of the head. These can so often be in need of help when there is infection such as in a catarrhal cold, or when the body is trying to throw out excessive waste and poisons from the body in the form of a mucous discharge. It has to be realized that infection in the respiratory tract occurs because the body's resistance is low and the waste matter in the system provides a suitable culture for the development of bacteria.

When massaging the big toe, first treat the top, which relates to the upper brain area. Then move to the all-important pituitary, the Master Gland. Stimulation by means of compression massage can assist in the regulation of the various processes of the secretions from the gland.

9. The Heart

The heart is a muscular organ which pumps the blood around the body, without ceasing, throughout the lifespan of the organism. Reflexology can be of very great use in helping various heart conditions and since it is given through the reflex in the left foot, or hand, it is quite safe to use.

The method of treatment varies according to the nature of the heart trouble. In cases where the whole body is in a state of low health with the tone of the muscles poor and flabby, the heart muscle will be in the same condition. General treatment over a period of time to improve the health will be needed, with special attention to the colon reflex.

Persistently poor circulation is one condition that will yield to our therapy. One patient of mine who had suffered with bad circulation all her life, with severe chilblains every winter, completely recovered and the chilblains went, never to return. Previously she had attended many health clinics without achieving any relief.

I have seen many old people suffering from acrocyanosis (blueness of the extremities) who have responded to the reflex treatment so well that the condition has gone after a few treatments as the circulation was stimulated. The general health of these old people improved to a remarkable degree.

Should someone suffer a severe heart attack, work as quickly as possible on the heart reflex in the left foot. There are many remarkable stories told of people who have fallen down, apparently dead, and who have been revived with deep massage given to the heart reflex. The impulse has been sufficient to stimulate the heart into action once more.

In cases of tachycardia, care should be taken to relax the patient by giving a full treatment to the feet, with special attention to the solar plexus, before giving massage to the heart reflex. If massage is given to the heart reflex first, it would probably increase the rapid pulse rate still further, so proceed with caution.

In long standing heart trouble amongst the elderly, give a general treatment on the reflexes with moderate pressure and only a few minutes on the heart reflex at first. The time can be increased gradually as the condition improves. I would ask those who decide to work on themselves, to start the work on the heart reflex gently at first. I know of a man who worked on his own feet and massaged for too long on the heart reflex. He gave himself a severe reaction and had to go to bed for a week.

A person with a weak heart may suffer severe distension of the colon, especially in the transverse where it starts to ascend to the splenic flexure. If a large amount of flatus should accumulate just under the heart and stomach, the condition may be a serious one, due to the poor peristalsis of the colon. Cases of heart failure have been known due to such a cause.

10. The Lungs

The lungs are organs of the respiratory system and are situated one on either side of the thoracic cavity. They are part of the means by which we live because they control the process of taking in air whereby the blood receives its oxygen. Also the lungs are one of the chief eliminating systems of the body. Without correct breathing the body cannot maintain good health. Severe tension has a serious effect upon the lungs, diminishing their ability to take in sufficient air and of course oxygen. In severe shock or tension the muscle of the diaphragm goes into spasm and prevents the lungs from expanding fully. Incorrect breathing and shallow breathing through tension over a long period will cause injury and is undoubtedly one of the contributory causes of asthma.

General treatment should be given on the foot below the eye and ear reflexes in the centre of the foot. A rather deep pressure is usually required, but as always the practitioner must be guided by the response of the patient. Also massage should be given on the top of the foot just below the base of the little toes and around the neck area of the big toes. Then the solar plexus reflex should be worked long enough to release fully any tension there. If tenderness is found which may be present even though the person is unaware of any trouble in the lungs, it could well be the result of earlier illnesses, even during childhood, such as pneumonia, pleurisy, or perhaps tuberculosis.

I know a man of about fifty who felt great discomfort when I worked on the left lung reflex. On questioning the patient I found that he had suffered from tuberculosis of the left lung when he was a small boy, and even though it was completely cured, the scar tissue still showed up as a tender area.

Asthma
This calls for a general treatment with extra massage to the pituitary, lung and solar plexus regions. Work also around the neck area of the big toe and between zones one and two, on the top of the foot which is on the side of the upper reflex

to the lung. Give attention to the adrenal gland by massaging the kidney reflex. The asthma patient always needs more cortisone to help the muscles of the lungs which are under strain. Thorough massage of the ileo-caecal valve reflex as well as those to the small intestines and colon is necessary to get the body to eliminate all waste matter and toxins. The heart reflex should also be treated.

If helping a patient with pneumonia, give treatment massage to the lung reflex, also the pituitary, solar plexus, and the heart reflex. Work on the ileo-caecal valve, too, but do not include the liver or intestines in the treatment until the patient is recovering from the acute stage.

11. The Kidneys

These glands lie on either side of the body in the second and third zones. They are delicate and complex mechanisms for secreting urine, water, salts, urea and acid bodies. The microscopic tubing in the cortex of a pair of kidneys is said to be very many miles long. From the kidneys, the two ureter tubes descend to the bladder. They are thin – about the size of a pencil – and are liable to pick up infections from the bladder if infection is present. The condition may travel up the ureter tubes endangering the kidneys, or the tubes may become partially blocked with sediment, mucus, and inflammation. In such cases the person will be suffering very great pain, passing urine with difficulty and at frequent intervals. The spread of the infection will be due to the feeble condition of the lymphatic glands in the groin which are not putting up a fight against the disorder.

Treatment by reflex massage should be given three times a week, if possible. In addition to the general massage, work on the pituitary, ureter, kidney and bladder reflexes should be carried out. But the very important areas for massage are the reflexes to the groin lymph nodes. The area over the foot and down around the ankle bones must be given concentrated massage with the thumbs and fingers

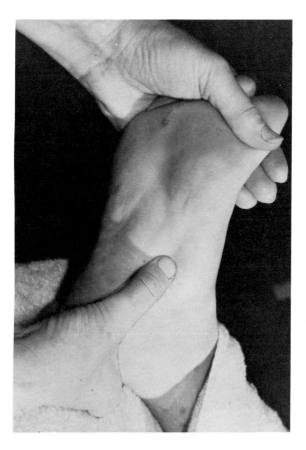

The reflex to the ureter tube

and then with the heel of the hand in order to stimulate the lymphatics into action.

My method of treating the urinary system is to start with massage on the bladder reflex, then to work slowly up the ureter tubes to the kidney and adrenal reflexes. Many remarkable recoveries are reported when reflexology is applied correctly.

Never forget to work on the kidney reflex for any kind of eye trouble.

It is possible to stimulate the kidney to eliminate stones by reflex massage in certain cases. These cases should be treated carefully. Massage should be given first to one kidney reflex until the stones are discharged. Then the process can be repeated on the other kidney area.

12. The Liver and Gall Bladder

The liver is the largest gland in the body and is to be found in all five zones on the right side of the medial line and the left lobe on zones one and two on the left side. But the reflex will show on the right foot, on the right of the solar plexus reflex.

The liver has many functions and the unusual characteristic of being able to reproduce a large part of itself if it has been surgically removed. It is an important area where many other organs are involved, and should be carefully checked when treating a new patient. Where there is severe congestion of the liver, the pain on pressure to the reflex will be extreme. Always remember to treat such a case with caution and do not give prolonged or heavy pressure at the first treatment, but explain to the sufferer that further treatments will be needed to clear the condition.

The reflex to the gall bladder lies to the left side of the liver reflex. In cases where gall stones are thought to be present, the area will show extreme tenderness. If there is a sluggish condition of the liver with an excess of bile, the patient will complain of liver pain. Treatment on the gall bladder reflex should give relief, but will have to be followed up by further treatments to bring back the healthy functioning of the liver and gall bladder. Do not forget that where there has been surgery for the removal of the gall bladder, there will be scar tissue present which will give rise to tension and discomfort which can also be relieved with massage.

Always remember that the whole length of the zone must be checked if the origin of the complaint is obscure, because pain may be referred from some other organ and manifest itself in a different part of the zone. One woman came to me who had had long-standing liver trouble. This was causing pain in the knee, lower leg and ankle. The pain was relieved by giving the massage to the liver reflex on the foot.

I had another case of a man who had suffered from continual pain at the back of the knee in the second zones for years. He had been under treatment from his doctors for the whole of the time. Osteopathic and physiotherapy treatment had also been given. The pain was unrelieved. On coming for treatment the man appeared to be in a low condition. The pain forced him to walk slowly and he could only walk upstairs one step at a time. He complained of eye trouble, and his sight seemed poor. He stated that the pain at the back of the knee joint persisted day and night. I gave him treatment and when I pressed the reflex to the liver, the pain was agonizing. Treatment was given in depth for as long as was advisable to the liver and gall bladder reflexes. A general treatment was also given to both feet and the eye reflex was found to be very sore. At the end of the session the man stood up and declared that the pain had left his knee. It was a definite case of referred pain along the zone from the liver to the knee, through the congestion of the liver. Treatments were continued for a while at weekly intervals. The man made a complete recovery from what had undoubtedly been severe congestion of the liver. The health of his eyes improved remarkably, also. It is worth noting that the trouble in the right eye, liver and knee (the pain occurred with greatest severity on the second and third zones of the knee) was in fact referred pain in the same zone. The man was a chef and his job involved doing a great deal of frying. It is not unreasonable to assume that he had eaten unwisely and had also absorbed a lot of oil through his skin with which his liver could not cope.

We must never forget that the whole body interacts one part with another. All parts link together to compose a complete structure. When dealing with a large vascular organ like the liver, remember that the muscle tone is very important. An unhealthy liver can seriously affect the whole circulation. Always ask those who first come for treatment about the history of the trouble in order to learn the nature of the disorder and its duration. The patient should be asked to note the reaction, if any, to the treatment, and whether a feeling of weariness or of well-being followed. A feeling of well-being points to a quick response by the body to the

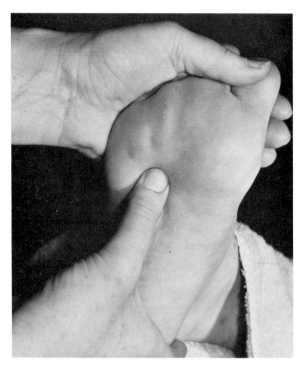

The liver and gall bladder area

stimulation given, and shows the return to a more normal condition.

In cases of gall stones this work is of great help, if the stones are small. Treatment should be given three times a week, if possible, with special work on the liver reflex. After about a fortnight the bile duct will probably be sufficiently dilated to allow the stones to pass through and into the duodenum, where they will be passed out of the body with the faeces. If the stones start to evacuate, the patient will complain of a sharp cutting pain across the waist line. When this occurs, **stop giving treatment** and allow nature to evacuate the stones. If the treatment is continued while the pain is severe, the patient will suffer increasing pain. Let nature take her own time. After the discomfort dies away, treatment can be continued if wished, but it is better to have an X-ray to check that all the stones have been cleared. I always request the patient to do so.

13. The Alimentary Canal

When giving treatment to a person for the first time, the organs of digestion must be checked for tenderness, when making a diagnosis. From the mouth to the anus disorders may occur. The stomach reflex, which is found on both feet just below the thyroid reflex, will often be tender if there is some form of disorder present. An indigestible meal will even show on the stomach reflex as tenderness to the area in half an hour after it has been eaten. Treatment should be given by careful massage working on both feet when it is found that trouble is present. Starting on the right foot on the stomach reflex, work in towards the middle of the foot downwards, to make contact with the area of the pylorus, which is the lower opening of the stomach, where food passes into the duodenum. An area in the lower part of the foot contains the reflexes to the small intestine, and massage should be given to the region shown on the chart at the back.

The all-important ileo-caecal valve, which separates the large and small intestine must always be checked carefully. If the valve is not functioning properly, it can be the cause of disorders in the sinuses, throat and lungs. If tenderness is found in the reflex, extra massage must be given. Always remember that constipation can be helped by our work and must be corrected. Long-standing constipation is the forerunner of many disorders. Massage carefully up the ascending colon and when you reach the hepatic flexure region, which is close to the liver reflex, be careful to work on it before starting to travel along the transverse colon. I find that many students are inclined to work too quickly, without giving sufficient massage where the ascending colon turns into the transverse colon. Give treatment on the transverse colon area first on the right foot and then on the left. As the practitioner approaches the part where the colon rises towards the hepatic flexure, the part may show great tenderness if the patient suffers from an unhealthy colon condition. The poor muscle tone will result in an accumulation of faecal matter in the area. Reflexology is of the greatest value in such cases through stimulation of the

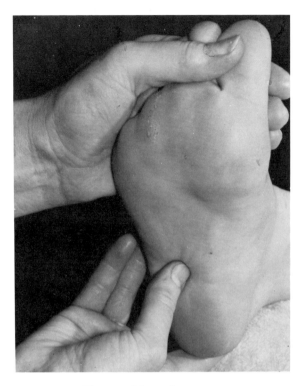

The small intestine area

peristalsis which will clear away the congestion. Always work up to the splenic flexure before going down the descending colon reflex. Here again soreness will be present if there is constipation. Much care must be given to the sigmoid reflex. It is in the sigmoid (S bend) that the trouble leading to malignancy will often be found in later life. Cross the lower part of the foot toward zone one, to the rectum reflex which is close to the bladder reflex.

For treating haemorrhoids work on the part adjoining the bladder reflex and also give deep massage up the back of the leg on either side of the Achilles tendon. If there is inflammation the response will be quite painful.

Always remember that many disorders of the heart, sinuses, ulceration of the legs and varicose veins may be caused by an unhealthy colon. The work of reflexology is invaluable in restoring the alimentary canal to good health.

14. The Lymphatic System

This is a circulatory system that works in close co-operation with blood circulation, yet is quite distinct from it. Throughout the body the lymph vessels are to be found linking the lymphatic glands.

The vessels between the glands have thin walls and are supplied with valves. The plasma in the blood flows out into the surrounding tissues, and there becomes the interstitial fluid, bringing nourishment to the cells and picking up waste matter. It is then collected by the lymphatic system and here it becomes the lymph which is carried to the glands for cleansing. It is finally poured into the right and left subclavian veins, after being purified.

The lymph is our great defender! Walls of these glands are placed in strategic positions in the body: around the head and neck, armpits and groin. These are placed to prevent infection from spreading throughout the body. The spleen, thymus and tonsils are all lymphatic glands. For all infections be sure that the correct area is checked and worked upon. Should the infection be in the teeth or tonsils, the massage should be given around the neck area of the big toe, especially on the inside of the toe moving across the top of the foot, working deeply into the roots of the little toes, which are the reflexes to the upper lymph glands. Apply extra massage to the spot between the third and fourth toes because the throat and Eustachian tube will be greatly stimulated in this way.

For an infection of the bladder or ureter tubes where there will be oedema of the ankles, work around the ankles with a deep but gentle massage. Very hard pressure will damage the tissues and cause rupturing of the peripheral capillaries. I have seen patches of broken red veins around the ankle due to rough handling – the sign of a bad practitioner! Help can be given to conditions of prostate and urinary weakness by working on the lymphatic reflexes.

The lymphatic glands of the underarm link with the breast, which is of course composed of lymph glands and vessels. To treat a breast disorder, massage across the top of the foot. Search carefully with the thumb or fingertips, as each breast covers all the zones — one to five. If a tender spot is found, question the patient as to whether she has a lump in the breast. Should a lump be present it will always be found in the same zone as the tender spot. Work carefully and thoroughly in the tender area and then continue the massage on the surrounding tissue for possible incipient lumps.

There are many cases on record of the successful dispersal of lumps from the breast following reflexology treatment. I have had great success in this field and my students too can quote many cases of disappearing congestion.

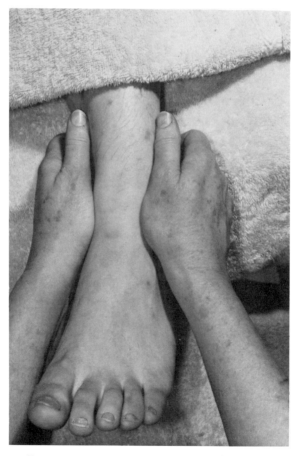

Deep massage on the lymphatic reflex area

There is such a close relationship between the reflexes of the foot and the breast that an injury to one may affect the other. An unusual story was told to me by a practitioner: a woman came to him with an abscess of the breast. When he tried to work upon the instep, which is of course the breast reflex, she was in agony. Thinking that the pain was more than should have been expected, he questioned her and found that a heavy crate of bottles had been dropped on her foot by a porter two or three months before. Evidently the bruising and damage to the tissues had been severe enough to cause the reflex impulse to work in reverse. Treatment was given and the woman recovered.

15. The Nervous System

The nerves of the body are messengers carrying impulses to and from the brain. It is not possible to go into the intricacy of their functions in this book. Suffice it to say that they play an all-important part in our work. As the reflex is massaged, the nerves carry the message to the brain, which in turn relays it to the organ linked to the reflex. When severe tension is present, the diaphragm is in a condition of spasm, and so unable to relax. This causes pressure on the lungs so that they cannot expand fully. As a result, the intake of oxygen drops, which lowers the ability of the body to revitalize itself. A remarkable change takes place as the tension is released and the circulation of the blood is increased.

Disorders of the Nerves
Sciatica is one of the prevalent nerve disorders. It is neuralgia of the sciatic nerve, quite often caused by pressure on the nerves in the spinal canal or a misaligned pelvis. There are other causes, such as pressure from the enlargement of an abdominal organ or again involvement with an arthritic condition. Treatment should be given across the heel of the foot on the sciatic loop working in with a

deep pressure because the skin of that area is hard and unyielding. Move along the edge of the heel to the Achilles tendon and then massage into the hollow area on either side of the tendon working up the leg for a few inches. Go slowly and note where the greatest tenderness is to be found. Use also the fingers and thumb to grasp the tendon and exert a slight pulling movement as you use the compression massage. Do not work up the leg or give massage on the thigh. Always treat from the foot area. Do not apply heat to the leg. In addition, always give a general treatment to both feet. Relax the solar plexus through massaging the reflex and give a lot of massage to the lymphatic area too.

Neuritis
The cause of neuritis is inflammation of the nerves, and the pain can be very acute. All movement is torture and will, if the attack is severe, incapacitate the patient. Never massage

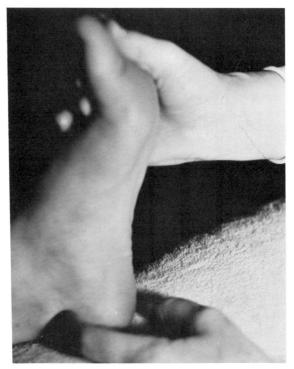

Massage on the sciatic reflex

the shoulder or use heat upon it. Instead, give careful massage to the reflexes of the feet. The big toe and the base of the little toe in zone five must have special attention. The neck area of the big toe should be worked upon and the toe rotated. Give a general treatment to both feet, and note any more areas. Use the cross reflexes, work the hip area on the feet, and deep massage applied directly on to the hip and thigh will help as well.

Herpes Zoster

This disorder is commonly known as shingles. It is a condition of inflamed nerves caused by a virus attacking the peripheral nerves. If requested to give help to someone suffering from shingles I would advise that no foot treatment be given while the disease is at the acute stage when the vesicles are present. The eruptions or blisters should be covered with plain talcum powder and lint to exclude the air. It is a nerve inflammation and the reflex massage may trigger off an acute attack of pain. I have seen this happen. Reflexology may be used with great advantage when the eruptions have healed. The patient will be depleted and in a low state and need all the help that can be given. Also it will prevent the unpleasant after effects of shingles known as causalgia, this is a persistent pain that will linger for years in the damaged nerves. I have been able to clear this condition even after years of distress, by using massage on the reflexes over a period of time.

16. The Skin

One of our important systems of elimination is the skin. It secretes water through the sweat glands carrying urea, salts, etc. The control of the heat regulating system of the body is done by the skin through the amount of perspiration evaporating from it. A healthy skin is soft, smooth and moist, with the glands and pores throwing out the waste products with the perspiration.

The work of reflexology is of great use in stimulating the movement of unwanted matter through the layers of the skin. In cases of obscure and recurring rashes it is very valuable.

Our bodies put up great resistance at first to any invading organism. Then, if they do not succeed in eliminating the toxins, or whatever the invaders may be, they are inclined to accept the condition, functioning and living alongside the alien substance. The first stage, where the body fights the invader, is known as the 'acute state'. The second is known as the 'chronic state' when the body accepts the situation. Our work in stimulating the reflexes encourages the body to resume its fight. The movements through the layers of skin are from below upwards. From the dermis to the epidermis. A poison may rest dormant in the tissues until stimulation brings the poisons to the surface, usually in the form of a skin rash.

One lady, who later became one of my early students, had been stung by a Portuguese Man of War jelly fish over a year before she came to see me. She had been quite ill following the attack, and was still suffering when I started to treat her. She said that she had patches of paralysis and numbness all over her legs, and also a recurring rash. When treatment was started the rash flared up in an acute form. She was a sensible woman and realized that this meant that the poison was being thrown out, so she continued with the treatment. In a short time the rash cleared, and so did all the other unpleasant symptoms to her great relief. She was so impressed with the wonderful way in which her trouble had been cleared that she decided to take the training herself.

The treatment was being given for very painful feet in addition to the primary condition. Both troubles responded to a full treatment on both feet once a week over a short period of time. Always remember that since the skin covers our bodies a general treatment to all the reflexes is most important. Give careful massage to the kidneys and adrenal gland reflexes for elimination and improved muscle tone. The lymphatics must not be forgotten, for they, too, play an important part in such cases.

17. The Female Reproductive System

Many of the disorders to be found in the uterus and ovaries yield to reflex massage in a remarkable way. Some of the more serious conditions are those of fibroid tumours, and cysts, yet many cases have been known where these have been dispersed both from the uterus and the ovaries. A case I had under my care was that of a young woman who had had one ovary removed a few years before. The trouble manifested in the other ovary with much pain, especially at the time of ovulation. The surgeon who attended her said she should have another operation for the removal of the ovary. Also her menstrual cycle was abnormal. Her periods occurred every twenty-one days accompanied by severe

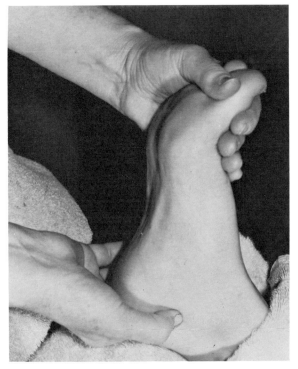

Position for massaging the uterus reflex

menstrual swelling of the body and breasts. Treatment was started weekly, and over a period of months the ovarian pain disappeared. The menstrual periods became normal and the premenstrual swelling became very much less. Today this patient is in excellent health.

Treatment for this case was given weekly with emphasis on the reflexes of the pituitary gland and thyroid gland, and also the reflexes of the uterus, ovaries and Fallopian tubes. A general treatment was always included. For tumours of the uterus a similar method of massage should be used. It is important that the woman has faith in the work and understands that about ten days after treatment she will in all probability have a discharge similar to a heavy period while nature is eliminating the congestion. When it is over, though, she should be free from any other trouble.

Reflexology is of great use in childbirth when the contractions are weak. One doctor reported a case to me of a woman who was in premature confinement. The contractions became very weak and finally died away. The doctor applied massage to the uterus reflex, and also to the back of the ankle on either side of the Achilles tendon. At once the contractions started vigorously again, and the child

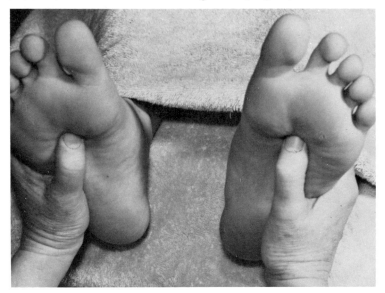

Breathing exercise to relax solar plexus

was safely delivered. One student has reported that she has had excellent results bringing about the birth of babies by using the massage on mothers who were overdue. In cases of delayed parturition, reflexology can avoid the need to have the baby artificially induced.

Amenorrhoea and scanty menstruation are conditions where reflex massage can be given with success. A course of treatment will usually correct the irregularity even when it has been present for a long time.

For women suffering from very heavy periods the feet should be worked upon throughout the month, but the treatment stopped during the actual flow because it may increase the discharge. It is not advisable to work on a woman in the early stages of pregnancy because there may be a weakness in the lining of the uterus which could cause a miscarriage.

There may be tenderness present on the ovary and uterus reflexes at any age. If hysterectomy has been performed, the resulting scar tissue will give rise to soreness on pressure.

Tension is always present where there is a disorder in a woman's reproductive system and treatment must always be given to the solar plexus reflex. The breathing exercise (mentioned on page 18) should be employed, the practitioner presses on the reflex while moving the feet in unison with the patient's slow breathing, and a complete release of tension is the result.

When treating cases similar to those that have been mentioned, never forget to work thoroughly on the pituitary and thyroid reflexes to restore the glandular balance. The uterus, ovaries and Fallopian tubes must receive massage, and also the back of the ankle on either side of the Achilles tendon. Whenever possible, a general treatment should be included.

18. The Prostate

Prostate trouble is a condition which responds very well to reflexology. Usually the improvement is apparent from the first treatment with the intervals between urination becoming progressively longer with each treatment. In cases of severe enlargement and discomfort, treatment should be given twice a week if possible and continued until the symptoms subside and the tension is relieved.

The reflex area for treatment is midway between the inner malleolus – or ankle – and the os calcis – or heel. Massage should be given in the area until the tenderness becomes less, if possible. Then deep massage should be given up the back of the heel on either side of the Achilles tendon.

For all disorders of the testicles the corresponding area on the outside of the foot should be treated. Massage should be given midway between the outer malleolus and the heel, and then carried over the ankle and around the lymphatic area to relieve congestion.

Early symptoms of incontinence should be treated in the area of the prostate reflex, and then forward along the foot, working down to the bladder reflex. This area should receive thorough massage. When giving general treatment over both feet, remember to always massage the adrenal glands and kidney reflexes. Stimulation of the adrenalin secretion is needed to increase the muscle tone of the sphincter muscle of the bladder. Good results should be obtained.

19. Arthritis

Arthritis is a progressive disease of the joints and it is usually divided into two classes: osteo-arthritis and rheumatoid-arthritis. There are variations of these two groups.

Arthritis may have different causes. Like all other disorders it is brought about by some condition which has thrown the body out of balance. Great physical strain and exposure to adverse conditions over a long period of time will induce the complaint. It is known that upon occasion arthritic subjects may have had too little synovial fluid in the joints and the condition may have been present even when they were quite young.

Faulty functioning of the intestines and the kidneys is a contributing cause. Poor nutrition plays a big part. Food deficiencies with inadequate vitamins and minerals prepare the way for disease. One of my patients who was an advanced arthritic told me that she had lived on an island for twenty years and for the whole time she had drunk only rain water. I have reason to believe that as all minerals would be lacking in pure rain water she was severely deprived of those trace elements which are so vital to health.

One cause of arthritis is an unhappy mind. The sufferer may have suppressed great sorrow, or be filled with resentment and hatred of circumstances or another person. Such a condition will throw the pituitary gland out of balance, which in turn will cause imbalance in all the other glands. The pituitary is very easily damaged in this way. I have a case in mind which will illustrate my belief. I knew a woman who was of fine physique, she had great enthusiasm for everything in which she believed, and she was an ardent vegetarian. She assured everyone she met that her good health was due to her diet, which no doubt it was. Unfortunately she was a possessive mother. One day her son, her only child, told her that he intended to leave home because he was going to marry. Her reaction to the news was one of intense anger because she was losing him, and of course she hated the girl for taking her son away from her. So powerful were the woman's emotions that in a few weeks the disharmony of her mind manifested itself in her body as severe arthritis. Even her healthy diet could not prevent the damage being done to her pituitary and all her endocrine glands. Quite soon she became crippled. At this time I moved away to another part of the country and lost sight of the poor woman. Perhaps she became reconciled to the marriage of the young couple, and if so maybe the harmony of her mind was restored by right thinking so that she recovered. I hope so.

The reflex treatment of arthritis is to help relieve the tension that has built up in the areas of inflammation around the joints and is causing the continual pain present in cases of arthritis. Through the reflexes of the feet we relax the affected areas. We also have to work to help the body to get rid of the accumulated poisons that lower the body's resistance and cause imbalance which is the origin of all disease. One patient was an old lady of ninety years of age who was suffering from severe spinal pain from arthritis which had followed a fall in her bath. A general treatment with special attention to the pituitary, thyroid and spinal reflexes was given once a week over a period of months, The pain in the spine disappeared, as well as a long standing disorder of the colon which had no doubt helped to induce the arthritis. The lady's general health improved greatly as well, to her delight.

Always treat for the improvement of the whole body by massage on all the reflexes of the feet to restore balance in all the functions. When giving treatment to an arthritic spine, in addition to a general massage on all the reflexes of the foot, give careful massage to the spinal reflex, working with persistance on all sore parts to help ease the tension. If after a few minutes the pain does not yield, pass on to the thyroid and adrenal reflexes, and also the sacro-iliac reflex. Remember that these cases will take time with perhaps three or four treatments needed before the pain begins to ease. There is no limit to the number of treatments that may

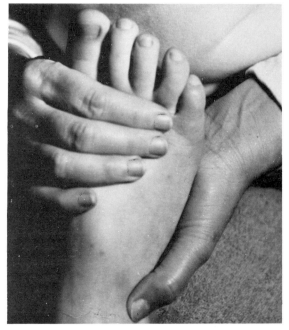

Position for massaging the sacro-iliac reflex

be given if the patient so wishes. In such cases there is always so much in the body needing the help of reflexology.

When the arthritic condition is present in the region of the pelvis, work with your finger and thumb deep into the tissues around the inner and outer maleolus (ankle). This part will always be sore. Extend your massage down towards the heel and up on either side of the Achilles tendon for the sciatic nerve reflex, which will always be involved in these cases.

Remember your cross reflexes, and for hip cases massage the shoulder reflex at the base of the little toe. Tell the patient to massage the reflexes in the hands, in between your visits, to help relieve the pain. Advise your patient to give direct massage to the shoulder as well. In cases of operations for hip joint replacement, where much laceration will have taken place due to the extensive surgery, a lot of help can be given by reflex massage to the shoulder. This will contribute to quicker healing of the tissues, and also help to cut down the tightening of the scar tissue which is being formed. In addition, any reflex massage that is given will alleviate shock resulting from the operation.

20. Case Histories

Head Pains (A Personal Account)

'I have been suffering for over twenty-two years with pains in my head, following an accident when I fractured my skull. This in turn had affected my spine and shoulder. However, in the last two years I also had radium treatment for carcinoma of the skin around the right eye, and this had increased my pains in the head, as the treatment had resulted in a blocked tearduct. My general condition was one of tiredness and exhaustion almost constantly, with high nervous tension. Having heard from a friend of reflexology I decided to give it a trial and on 5 July 1973, made an appointment to see Mrs Bayly. For purposes of record I am keeping these notes of my progress during the treatment.

5 July 1973. Initial treatment. Told Mrs Bayly of head pains but only very briefly. However, she started on my feet and I

was amazed to find how accurately she was able to pinpoint where I get pains, *i.e.*, spine, shoulder, sinus and solar plexus. The sinus reflexes were particularly painful as were also those of the lungs. After about half-an-hour the treatment was finished. I felt extremely calm and relaxed, something I had not felt for ages.

By Monday of the 9 July I had quite a bit of sneezing but felt so energetic and alive it was quite remarkable. My eyes, instead of being puffed up with congestion as formerly, were much larger and brighter. I had, however, quite a lot of pain in the region of the solar plexus, the area which was always affected by tension — a feeling almost like *sand* instead of blood — very uncomfortable. Coughing a lot and expectorating which suggests to me a clearing of the obstruction in the lungs.

Am so *calm* at work I can't believe it. Am working very well and efficiently without the awful feeling of panic that has been assailing me lately.

Thursday, 12 July 1973. Toes extremely painful, when I first get up, but get better as I walk about.

Thursday, 12 July (evening). Further treatment from Mrs Bayly. Some areas more painful than others. However, as before went home feeling very cheerful and relaxed.

Friday, 13 July. Awoke feeling *terribly* tired and deep-seated intense pain behind both eyes. Really intense pain, similar to pain experienced when a poultice is applied to a boil. Feel awful and wonder how I can face the day's work. Pain continued and sleep almost impossible as worse lying flat. Awoke Saturday morning and pain so bad in eyes, head and behind ear, and left of neck, decided I must get medical treatment. Went to Doctor in morning who arranged an urgent appointment for me at Southend Hospital for Monday.

Late Saturday afternoon the pain started to go, but *thick* yellow discharge coming from eye. Shall see how I feel Monday. If pain gone should cancel hospital appointment because I now feel that this could be result of Mrs Bayly's treatment which is clearing all congestion in the head.

Certainly apart from these head pains I feel very well, and have a lot of energy. I *look* better, too, and have lost that awful *white* look I used to have in morning. Feel cheerful and calm in spite of pain in head and eyes.

Sunday. Pain gone completely from head — eye (left) still discharging yellow pus and very watery. The energy flow is fantastic! Up at 7 o'clock and working right through cleaning house, windows, gardening, taking dog for walk until 2 p.m. Feel so cheerful and alert. I feel as I used to feel when I was 30! To think only a few weeks ago I would have been exhausted by 10 a.m. and have had to keep sitting down! I shall stay faithful to my intuitive belief that reflexology can help my condition and cancel hospital appointment tomorrow.'

This lady lived some distance from London, and found it impossible to make the journey for treatments because her son was away. She wrote how greatly improved her condition was on 20 July 1973, and nearly two months later she wrote: 'Only *one* headache in the last four weeks. Isn't it wonderful!' She reported that she had gone to the hospital about her eye 'although I felt I was wasting their time as after that heavy discharge it was better' and was told that apart from a little conjunctivitis it was quite well. The therapy 'has done me so much good!' she exclaimed.

Back Injury
The patient was a man of forty-four years of age who had been a famous cricketer. When he first came to me he was both stiff and slow in movement and his complexion was of a very poor colour.

The history of the case was that he had injured his back, for which a great deal of orthodox treatment had been given without result. He had been X-rayed and was told that the hips were showing incipient arthritis and the general stiffness was due to the condition.

Treatment was started and many very tender reflexes were found. The feet were unyielding at first, but they became more supple after a few treatments. The right leg was the one affected by the back condition and the usual area of numbness (analgesia) was found on the top of the foot. The foot was lacking in muscle tone and the toes had very little strength when the patient was asked to push against my hand. *But the reflex to the hips showed no tenderness* as one would expect if the hips were arthritic. The sciatic stirrup down either side of the Achilles tendon and under the heel was tender, but this condition gradually improved.

I believed that the general stiffness had been brought about by excessive tension over the years. No doubt he had played in tension and continued in tension, both sleeping and waking. This, I believe, had resulted in the glands of the body gradually slowing down due to a diminished blood supply.

Special attention was given to all the gland reflexes and advice given on relaxing exercises. Gradually the patient's strength returned. The stiffness slowly disappeared, and his colour improved. The numbed area on the foot receded and with exercise the foot and toes became stronger. Soon he was able to enjoy a two-day visit to a golf course by the sea without pain or discomfort. A few weeks later he was able to take his team to the Far East to attend a big cricket match organized for charity.

Sinus Trouble

A lady of mature years who was suffering with a chronic infection of the sinuses was recommended to come to me for treatment. The attacks were so severe that she ran a temperature and felt so very ill that she did not risk going out during the winter. The trouble had also spread to her eyes through the infected tear ducts. The disorder was of some years standing and was causing the lady great distress.

On examining her feet I found that the whole of her reflexes were in an extremely tender condition, especially the colon reflex. This was definitely a case of long standing constipation, and a slow poisoning of the body had been taking place. The ileo-caecal valve had been unable to cope and the poisons had been thrown up into the sinuses.

The feet were so painful that only the lightest pressure could be given at first. The reflex to the pituitary and the small toes in the sinus reflex area were given concentrated treatment, together with the reflex to the lungs and the solar plexus to ease the severe tension. Massage to the liver and small intestines together with persistent work on the colon reflex was given at each visit. I would traverse the colon reflex two or three times, and then work in reverse from the reflex of the rectum and along the whole of the colon reflex to the caecum. Very gradually the extreme tenderness grew less, and the pain in the sinuses improved as the poison was eliminated. The eyes were more slow to improve, but they too finally cleared. The lady's general health became so much improved that the following winter she was able to live a normal life and go about freely without a recurrence of the trouble. In these cases a little advice on diet to help the normal functioning of the intestines is always given, to enable the body to recover from long standing abuse. The lady's health is now excellent.

Cerebral Haemorrhage

Cerebral haemorrhage, or stroke, is a condition where the blood vessels in the brain rupture causing a haemorrhage to take place. The cause may be high blood pressure and hardening of the arteries (arterio-sclerosis). Severe tension in the solar plexus caused by anger or emotional distress can upset the body's systems and lead to a stroke. Unusual exertion or shock may provoke the condition.

We all know that the controls of the body cross as they leave the brain. If haemorrhage has taken place on one side, the paralysis will be apparent on the other side of the body. The reflex impulse does not cross in this way and we work on both feet equally.

If you have to treat a person who has just suffered a stroke, work on them as quickly as possible. I have found the response to be most remarkable. By working on the brain reflex in both big toes as well as other important areas you will be able to assist the blood circulation considerably. This helps to prevent clotting and reduces the pressure of the haemorrhage in an enclosed area.

Prompt reflexology helps the circulation to function and the blood to supply oxygen to the brain cells, so that not only will the patient show signs of recovery but paralysis will be prevented. A friend of mine in the United States saved her husband from becoming an invalid by these means. He was a high powered executive in spite of poor health and the fact that he had only one kidney. One evening when they were alone in their home he had a stroke and there were no doctors available. The wife had some knowledge of reflexology although she had not been trained. Very quickly she pulled off his shoes and commenced massage upon the feet. She gave a thorough treatment. The next day their reflex practitioner came along and again treated the patient. It was two days before the doctor arrived. When he saw the man's condition he exclaimed, 'You have performed a miracle! By working at once on his feet you have kept the blood circulating through the brain so the cells have been able to receive the necessary oxygen. I am happy to tell you that he will not suffer any paralysis.' This proved to be the case and within a few weeks the man returned to his busy office life.

In one case I was able to treat an elderly man almost immediately after his stroke. When I arrived he looked extremely ill and his colour was poor. He had lost control of his speech, and his eyes could not focus. Treatment was given as follows. Both big toes were massaged for the brain area and the pituitary reflex also the cervical reflexes to prevent tension building at the back of the neck. Massage was given to the heart reflex to increase circulation, and to the reflex to the solar plexus to quieten the patient. At the end of twenty minutes the blueness had left his face and he was able to speak to me. He focussed his eyes on my face without difficulty.

When treating such a case please remember what the patient is experiencing. It must be a terrifying ordeal to know that you cannot move or speak. Much can be done to help by talking soothingly while giving the treatment. This I always do because the ability to hear is the last sense to be lost. Even by just telling the patient that you are going to help him to recover, you are doing just that.

Here let me say again how very wrong it is for people to stand near to and talk about the sick person. The ability to hear is often more acute when very ill. I have even seen nurses, I am sorry to say, commit this very grave error, by talking and discussing the illness as though the patient was an inanimate object instead of a living person.

In cases where the stroke has occurred some time before, work on the reflexes will be necessary for some time. Very good results will be obtained if massage is given consistently over a period of time. One case told to me by a colleague was of a woman who had suffered three strokes and is an example of the helpfulness of delayed reflexology. The woman had had her last stroke twenty months before, and had been left paralysed in the arm and leg. She needed to be helped whenever she went from one room to another. Treatment was started weekly. Her husband was shown how to work on her feet between the visits of the practitioner. She made such a good recovery that she was able to travel on a bus alone.

Poor Health in Old Age

A lady of seventy-nine was suffering from acrocyanosis of hands and feet. This was accompanied by a tremor and a general appearance of weakness. Treatment was started at weekly intervals and gradually her health improved. The blue colour of her hands and feet entirely disappeared.

The patient said that she had been suffering from a discharge of blood from the bladder prior to receiving reflexology treatment. Her doctor assured her that nothing could be done to help this trouble at her age. As treatment proceeded the slow haemorrhage gradually ceased from the bladder, due to the improvement in her general health. The regular massage of the lymphatics had no doubt overcome the chronic infection by stimulating them to fight the condition.

The general appearance of the lady greatly improved. She walked more quickly and her thinking powers became more alert. Her gratitude was overwhelming since her doctor had repeatedly told her that he could do nothing for her at her age.

A lady in her early seventies was in a very low state of health. She had always been delicate. She was almost totally deaf in her right ear as the result of a mastoid operation as a child. There was a spinal curvature requiring a surgical corset. The sight of the right eye had also gone. The lungs were in a poor condition due to a neglected attack of pneumonia about ten years before I met her. There was very little expansion of the lungs when breathing. The sound of bubbling mucus was heard when she attempted to take a deeper breath. Her hands and feet were badly cyanosed. The kidneys and bladder were functioning badly. As in the previous case there was a discharge of blood from the bladder. Examinations in hospital confirmed that the haemorrhage was definitely coming from the urinary tract.

Treatment was started and continued over a period of months. The improvement was steady but consistent. The hands and feet became normal in colour. The right side of the body, which had always been weak, became stronger and the right foot ceased to give pain. Recommended simple breathing exercises were undertaken and the breathing improved considerably. Also the haemorrhaging from the bladder ceased. The patient became more upright and breathing continued to improve. She became brighter, stronger and no longer depressed. She also looked several years younger.

Disseminated Sclerosis

A lady of about thirty years old came to me for treatment. She said that she had been diagnosed as a sclerosis case twenty months before when she had attended hospital where she was described as a typical sufferer of the disease in its early stages. Her symptoms were numbness of the feet and legs, and a feeling of tightness around the hips.

At the beginning of her treatment I was aware of the energy flow being absent but at the end I felt there was a change. I asked her if, on her visit to hospital, the specialist had drawn a sharp instrument along her foot. She replied that he had done so but she had not felt anything. I then drew my thumb-nail down her foot and she responded sharply and was amazed that she had felt it.

Her treatments were continued, at first twice a week and then once weekly over a period of two or three months. At the end of this time the numbness had left her legs and feet and she was feeling very well indeed.

Now, it is known that remissions occur sometimes in these cases, but if it were a remission, it was a very good one.

Parkinson's Disease

A man aged seventy-seven had been diagnosed as a Parkinson's case the morning he was brought to me. He had all the usual symptoms and was very slow and stiff. He had to be helped into the reclining chair. Treatments were given at first twice a week, then once a week. He responded well, gradually regained strength and became more alert. Finally the stiffness left his shoulders and he was able to move quite freely. He took up his normal life again. He died in his eighties without a recurrence of the trouble.

Treatment:
When treating any type of paralysis, I always give extra massage to the big toe area and work very thoroughly over the top of the toe and then gradually down the sides so that the whole brain reflexes receive stimulation. Then I give consistent pressure around the neck area of the toe, especially on the cervical reflex. Continue down the spine slowly giving a deep but careful pressure. On reaching the coccyx give a searching massage and note the reaction, if any.

A general treatment of the feet should then be given, questioning the patient on the degree of sensitivity or areas of numbness experienced. Before the end of the massage the head and spine areas may again receive, briefly, further treatment.

I endeavour to see the patient twice a week until a good response to the work has been established. Then once a week will be sufficient, but be prepared for recovery to be slow.

Extreme Bruising

Some little while ago I was asked to see a lady who had fallen on some stone steps. She was at the time carrying parcels in both hands so that she fell forward with full force on her face. The blow against the steps fractured the zygoma (cheek bone). All the flesh on the area above the fracture was terribly damaged, but nothing could be done surgically. It just had to heal itself. The most painful thing was that the damaged tissues adhered to the bone. This caused much tension and distress.

I treated for shock by working on the solar plexus and the endocrine gland reflexes. For the injury itself, massage was given to the area corresponding to the face on the inside of the two big toes. Then a very thorough general treatment was given to both feet. There was some relief felt even from the first treatment. On subsequent treatments the dark bruised area of the cheek grew less each time the treatment was given. The lady made a complete recovery.

Foot Trouble

A man who was sent to me for treatment had been suffering from great pain in his feet for twenty years. In fact he had

been in trouble with his feet ever since he was in the Italian
Army during the war. He was a very young lad at the time,
and marching in heavy boots had been torture for him. I
found the feet very stiff and hard with very little movement,
but the skin was soft. The muscle tone was very poor. On
being relaxed with massage the feet became more pliable.
On the left foot the arch had dropped. Pain was found in the
spinal reflexes due to an injury through lifting a piano some
years ago.

Treatment was given on both feet with extra treatment on
the solar plexus area. Extra manipulation followed to help
the feet regain more flexibility. A small pad of adhesive felt
was applied to both feet to help the weak arches and correct
the posture. Great relief was felt from the first treatment.
After two or three visits he declared that he was no longer in
pain for the first time in all those years.

Arthritis

One practitioner in Belfast, who is very successful, told me
of a case of an elderly man who was suffering from a chronic
and severe condition of arthritis of the knee which prevented
him from walking upstairs and kept him awake at night.
Treatment was given every week for nearly three months
without change, then the condition yielded to the treatment,
the knee ceased to be painful, secondary conditions such as
catarrh also improved. The man was so delighted and felt so
fit that he telephoned his daughter to expect him for
Christmas. This practitioner says that reflexology and
nothing else restored the body to its natural balance, for the
patient refused to take any other treatment. This is a clear
case of patient work on a chronic case. This practitioner
suggests that our motto should be 'Press on regardless'.

Kidney Troubles

Another interesting case was told to me by a student in
Geneva. She had treated a man who had been suffering
from a serious and long-standing kidney complaint. He also
complained of pains in his feet and declared that they were
getting shorter. On examination it was found that the soles
of the feet showed hard and contracted tissue over the
kidney, ureter tube and bladder reflexes. After a course of
reflexology the kidney condition improved and the

contracted tissue relaxed and disappeared.

Eczema and Asthma
A lady in Wales asked for help for her daughter of five and a half who had suffered from infantile eczema almost from birth and asthma from the age of two. I recommended her to a very good practitioner who lived in North Wales about forty miles away. She took the child to this lady once a week. The treatment was very successful.

Index

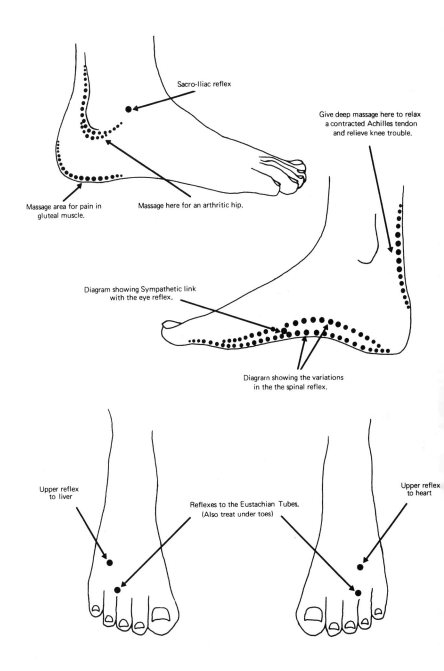

Sacro-Iliac reflex

Give deep massage here to relax
a contracted Achilles tendon
and relieve knee trouble.

Massage area for pain in
gluteal muscle.

Massage here for an arthritic hip.

Diagram showing Sympathetic link
with the eye reflex.

Diagram showing the variations
in the the spinal reflex.

Upper reflex
to liver

Reflexes to the Eustachian Tubes.
(Also treat under toes)

Upper reflex
to heart

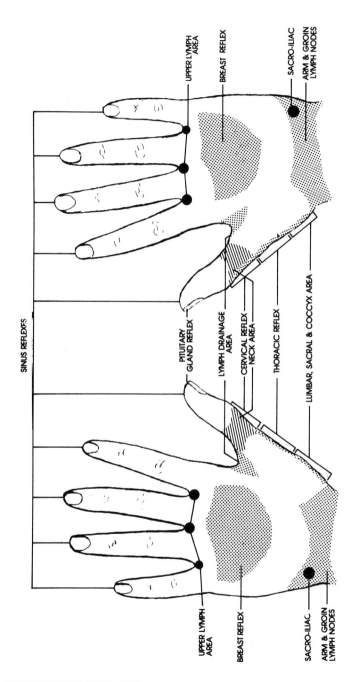

REFLEXOLOGY, HAND REFLEX CHART
Designed and Published by Doreen E. Bayly
© 1973

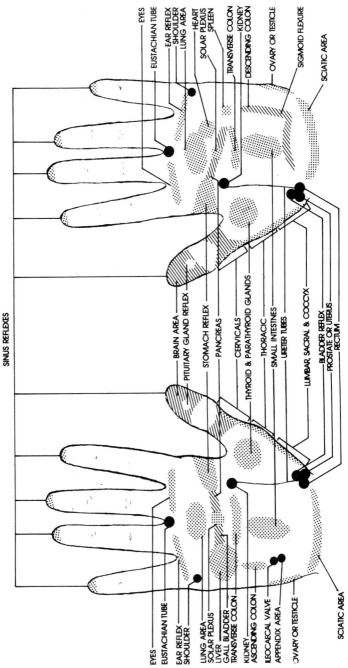

SINUS REFLEXES

EYES
EUSTACHIAN TUBE
EAR REFLEX
SHOULDER
LUNG AREA
HEART
SOLAR PLEXUS
SPLEEN
TRANSVERSE COLON
KIDNEY
DESCENDING COLON
OVARY OR TESTICLE
SIGMOID FLEXURE
SCIATIC AREA

BRAIN AREA
PITUITARY GLAND REFLEX
STOMACH REFLEX
PANCREAS
CERVICALS
THYROID & PARATHYROID GLANDS
THORACIC
SMALL INTESTINES
URETER TUBES
LUMBAR, SACRAL & COCCYX
BLADDER REFLEX
PROSTATE OR UTERUS
RECTUM

EYES
EUSTACHIAN TUBE
EAR REFLEX
SHOULDER
LUNG AREA
SOLAR PLEXUS
LIVER
GALL BLADDER
TRANSVERSE COLON
KIDNEY
ASCENDING COLON
ILEOCAECAL VALVE
APPENDIX AREA
OVARY OR TESTICLE
SCIATIC AREA